Plant-Based Alimentation

You Can't Go Wrong With This Win-Win Cookbook for You and the Planet

The Green Solution

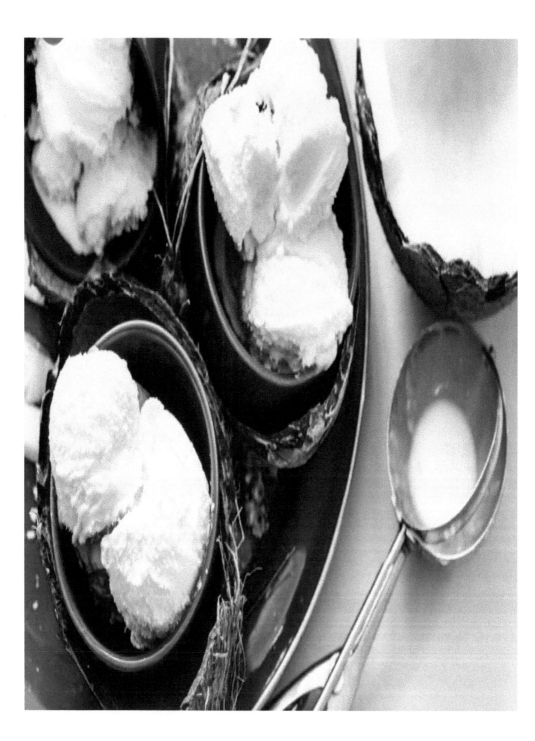

Table of Contents

INTRODUCTION

A plant-based diet is a diet consisting mostly or entirely of plant-based foods with no animal products or artificial ingredients. While a plant-based diet avoids or has limited animal products, it is not necessarily vegan. This includes not only fruits and vegetables, but also nuts, seeds, oils, whole grains, legumes, and beans. It doesn't mean that you are vegetarian or vegan and never eat meat, eggs, or dairy.

Vegetarian diets have also been shown to support health, including a lower risk of developing coronary heart disease, high blood pressure, diabetes, and increased longevity.

Plant-based diets offer all the necessary carbohydrates, vitamins, protein, fats, and minerals for optimal health, and are often higher in fiber and phytonutrients. However, some vegans may need to add a supplement to ensure they receive all the nutrients required.

Who says that plant-based diets are limited or boring? There are lots of delicious recipes that you can use to make mouthwatering, healthy, plant-based dishes that will satisfy your cravings. If you're eating these plant-based foods regularly, you can maintain a healthy weight without obsessing about calories and avoid diseases that result from bad dietary habits.

Benefits of a Plant-Based Diet

Eating a plant-based diet improves the health of your gut so you are better able to absorb the nutrients from food that support your immune system and reduce inflammation. Fiber can lower cholesterol and stabilize blood sugar, and it's great for good bowel management.

- **A Plant-Based Diet May Lower Your Blood Pressure**
  High blood pressure, or hypertension, can increase the risk for health issues, including heart disease, stroke, and type 2 diabetes and reduce blood pressure and other risky conditions.

- **A Plant-Based Diet May Keep Your Heart Healthy**
  Saturated fat in meat can contribute to heart issues when eaten in excess, so plant-based foods can help keep your heart healthy.

- **A Plant-Based Diet May Help Prevent Type 2 Diabetes**
  Animal foods can increase cholesterol levels, so eating a plant-based diet filled with high-quality plant foods can reduce the risk of developing type 2 diabetes by 34 percent.

- **Eating a Plant-Based Diet Could Help You Lose Weight**
  Cutting back on meat can help you to maintain a healthy weight because a plant-based diet is naturally satisfying and rich in fiber.

- **Following a Plant-Based Diet Long Term May Help You Live Longer**
  If you stick with healthy plant-based foods your whole body will be leaner and healthier, allowing you to stay healthy and vital as you age.

- **A Plant-Based Diet May Decrease Your Risk of Cancer**
  Vegetarians have an 18 percent lower risk of cancer compared to non-vegetarians. This is because a plant-based diet is rich of fibers and healthy nutrients.

- **A Plant-Based Diet May Improve Your Cholesterol**
  High cholesterol can lead to fatty deposits in the blood, which can restrict blood flow and potentially lead to heart attack, stroke, heart disease, and many other problems. A plant-based diet can help in maintaining healthy cholesterol levels.

- **Ramping Up Your Plant Intake May Keep Your Brain Strong**
  Increased consumption of fruits and vegetables is associated with a 20 percent reduction in the risk of cognitive impairment and dementia. So plant foods can help protect your brain from multiple issues.

What to Eat in Plant-Based Diets

Fruits: Berries, citrus fruits, pears, peaches, pineapple, bananas, etc.

Vegetables: Kale, spinach, tomatoes, broccoli, cauliflower, carrots, asparagus, peppers, etc.

Starchy vegetables: Potatoes, sweet potatoes, butternut squash, etc.

Whole grains: Brown rice, rolled oats, farro, quinoa, brown rice pasta, barley, etc.

Healthy fats: Avocados, olive oil, coconut oil, unsweetened coconut, etc.

Legumes: Peas, chickpeas, lentils, peanuts, black beans, etc.

Seeds, nuts, and nut butters: Almonds, cashews, macadamia nuts, pumpkin seeds, sunflower seeds, natural peanut butter, tahini, etc.

Unsweetened plant-based milks: Coconut milk, almond milk, cashew milk, etc.

Spices, herbs, and seasonings: Basil, rosemary, turmeric, curry, black pepper, salt, etc.

Condiments: Salsa, mustard, nutritional yeast, soy sauce, vinegar, lemon juice, etc.

Plant-based protein: Tofu, tempeh, plant-based protein sources or powders with no added sugar or artificial ingredients.

Beverages: Coffee, tea, sparkling water, etc.

What Not to Eat in Plant-Based Diets

Fast food: French fries, cheeseburgers, hot dogs, chicken nuggets, etc.

Added sugars and sweets: Table sugar, soda, juice, pastries, cookies, candy, sweet tea, sugary cereals, etc.

Refined grains: White rice, white pasta, white bread, bagels, etc.

Packaged and convenience foods: Chips, crackers, cereal bars, frozen dinners, etc.

Processed vegan-friendly foods: Plant-based meats like; Tofurkey, faux cheeses, vegan butters, etc.

Artificial sweeteners: Equal, Splenda, Sweet'N Low, etc.

Processed animal products: Bacon, lunch meats, sausage, beef jerky, etc.

Day 1:

Breakfast (304 calories)

- 1 serving Berry-Kefir Smoothie

A.M. Snack (95 calories)

- 1 medium apple

Lunch (374 calories)

- 1 serving Green Salad with Pita Bread & Hummus

P.M. Snack (206 calories)

- 1/4 cup dry-roasted unsalted almonds

Dinner (509 calories)

- 1 serving Beefless Vegan Tacos
- 2 cups mixed greens
- 1 serving Citrus Vinaigrette

Day 2:

Breakfast (258 calories)

- 1 serving Cinnamon Roll Overnight Oats
- 1 medium orange

A.M. Snack (341 calories)

- 1 cup low-fat plain Greek yogurt
- 1 medium peach
- 3 Tbsps slivered almonds

Lunch (332 calories)

- 1 serving Thai-Style Chopped Salad with Sriracha Tofu

P.M. Snack (131 calories)

- 1 large pear

Dinner (458 calories)

- 1 serving Mexican Quinoa Salad

Day 3:

Breakfast (258 calories)

- 1 serving Cinnamon Roll Overnight Oats
- 1 medium orange

A.M. Snack (95 calories)

- 1 medium apple

Lunch (463 calories)

- 1 serving Thai-Style Chopped Salad with Sriracha Tofu
- 1 large pear

P.M. Snack (274 calories)

- 1/3 cup dried walnut halves
- 1 medium peach

Dinner (419 calories)

- 1 serving Eggs in Tomato Sauce with Chickpeas & Spinach
- 1 1-oz. slice whole-wheat baguette

BONUS PLANT-BASED RECIPES

Steamed Homemade Asian Brussels Sprouts

Servings: 8

Preparation Time: 20 minutes

Per Serving: Calories 137, Total Fat 11g, Saturated Fat 2g, Total Carbs 8g, Net Carbs 6g, Protein 4g, Sugar: 3g, Fiber: 2g, Sodium: 137mg, Potassium: 205mg, Phosphorus: 63mg

Ingredients:

- 8 teaspoons soy sauce
- 2 cups of water
- 3 cups Brussels sprouts, thinly sliced
- Salt to taste
- 4 tablespoons chopped peanuts, toasted
- 4 tablespoons sesame oil
- 4 teaspoons rice vinegar

Procedure:

1. First of all, pour water into the Instant Pot and place a steamer basket or trivet inside.
2. Take a heat-proof dish, mix all ingredients except for the peanuts.
3. Then toss to coat the Brussels sprouts with the ingredients.
4. Place the dish with the Brussels sprouts on the trivet.
5. Now close the lid and set the vent to the Sealing position.

6. Press the Steam button and cook for 10 minutes.
7. Do natural pressure release to open the lid.
8. Finally, garnish with toasted peanuts before serving.

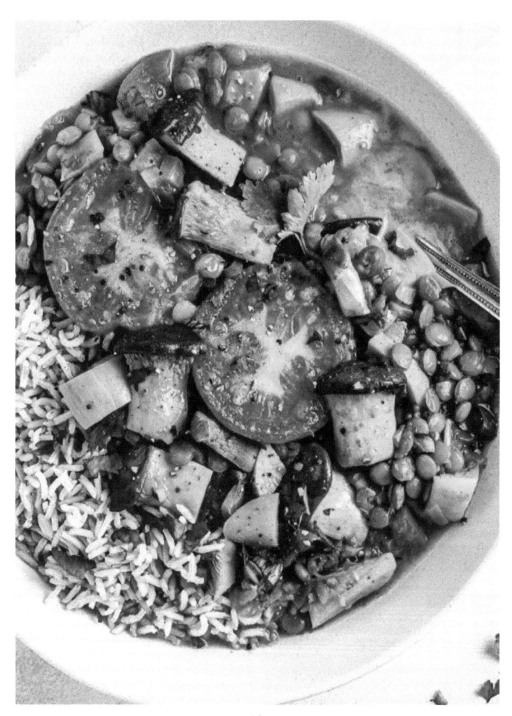

Rice, Mushroom & Vegetable Curry

Servings: 12

Preparation Time: 35 minutes

Per Serving: Calories 174, Total Fat 10g, Saturated Fat 2g, Total Carbs 23g, Net Carbs 15g, Protein 7g, Sugar: 7g, Fiber: 8g, Sodium: 147mg, Potassium: 968mg, Phosphorus: 450mg

Ingredients:

- 2 bunches of fresh coriander, chopped
- 2 fresh chilies, chopped
- 2 teaspoons turmeric powder
- 2 teaspoons fenugreek seeds
- 2 teaspoons black mustard seeds
- 2 tablespoons olive oil
- 4 cloves of garlic, minced
- 2 onions, chopped
- Salt and pepper to taste
- 1 cup of water
- 2 teaspoons curry powder
- 1 pound mixed mushrooms sliced
- 1 pound of mixed vegetables
- 1 cup brown basmati rice
- 2 28-ounce coconut milk

Procedure:

1. First of all, press the Sauté button on the Instant Pot and heat the oil.
2. Sauté the garlic and onion for a minute.
3. Stir in the chili, turmeric powder, fenugreek seeds, mustard seeds, and curry powder.
4. Then stir for another minute or until toasted.
5. Stir in the mushrooms and stir for 3 minutes or until wilted.
6. Now stir in the rest of the ingredients except for the coriander.
7. Close the lid and do not seal the vent.
8. Then press the Rice button and cook using the preset cooking time.
9. Once cooked, stir in the coriander last.

Smoked Vegetable Chili

Servings: 10

Preparation Time: 40 minutes

Per Serving: Calories 586, Total Fat 4g, Saturated Fat 0.7g, Total Carbs 126g, Net Carbs 108g, Protein 15g, Sugar: 14g, Fiber: 18g, Sodium: 123mg, Potassium: 3131mg, Phosphorus: 426mg

Ingredients:

- 2 tablespoons olive oil
- 4 onions, chopped
- 16 small jacket potatoes
- 2 bunches of fresh coriander, chopped
- Salt and pepper to taste
- 2 cups of water
- 2 teaspoons cumin seeds
- 4 teaspoons smoked paprika
- 6 mixed color peppers, seeded and chopped
- 6 large tomatoes, chopped
- 4 teaspoons cocoa powder
- 2 tablespoons peanut butter
- 2 fresh chilies, chopped
- 4 sweet potatoes, peeled and cubed

Procedure:

1. Firstly, press the Sauté button on the Instant Pot and heat the oil.

2. Sauté the onions and cumin until fragrant.
3. Then stir in the paprika, cocoa powder, peanut butter, chili, peppers, tomatoes, and potatoes.
4. Now season with salt and pepper and pour in water.
5. Close the lid and set the vent to the Sealing position.
6. After that, press the Meat/Stew button and cook using the preset cooking time.
7. Do natural pressure release.

Easy Sicilian Aubergine Stew

Servings: 10

Preparation Time: 30 minutes

Per Serving: Calories 161, Total Fat 10g, Saturated Fat 1g, Total Carbs 9g, Net Carbs 7g, Protein 10g, Sugar: 3g, Fiber: 2g, Sodium: 131mg, Potassium: 323mg, Phosphorus: 99mg

Ingredients:

- 4 large tomatoes, chopped
- 2 tablespoons caper
- 4 tablespoons olive oil
- 2 small onions, chopped
- 6 cloves of garlic, minced
- 1 cup couscous
- salt and pepper to taste
- 6 cups of water
- 2 large aubergines, chopped
- 2 tablespoons flaked almonds
- 16 green olives, pitted
- 2 tablespoons red wine vinegar

Procedure:

1. Firstly, press the Sauté button and heat the olive oil.
2. Sauté the onion and garlic until fragrant.
3. Then stir in the aubergine and tomatoes for three minutes until slightly wilted.

4. Add the capers, olives, red wine vinegar, and couscous.
5. Now season with salt and pepper to taste and pour water.
6. Close the lid and set the vent to the Sealing position.
7. After that, press the Meat/Stew button and adjust the cooking time to 20 minutes.
8. Do natural pressure release.
9. Once the lid is open, sprinkle with flaked almonds.

Aubergine Dip

Servings: 4

Preparation Time: 20 minutes

Per Serving: Calories 102, Total Fat 4g, Saturated Fat 0.5g, Total Carbs 18g, Net Carbs: 9 g, Protein 3g, Sugar: 10g, Fiber: 9g, Sodium: 66mg, Potassium: 662mg, Phosphorus: 72mg

Ingredients:

- 2 tablespoons extra-virgin olive oil
- Juice from 1 lemon
- 1 teaspoon smoked paprika
- 2 large aubergines
- 2 cloves of garlic, minced
- 2 fresh green chilies, minced
- Salt and pepper to taste

Procedure:

1. First, pour water into the Instant Pot and place a trivet or steamer basket inside.
2. Place the aubergines inside.
3. Then close the lid and set the vent to the Sealing position.
4. Now press the Steam button and cook for 10 minutes.
5. Do natural pressure release.

6. After that, remove the aubergine from the Instant Pot and allow it to cool.
7. Once cooled, peel the aubergine and place it in a food processor.
8. Add the rest of the ingredients. Pulse until smooth.
9. Finally, serve with crackers.

Homemade Vegetables in Tomatoes

Servings: 8

Preparation Time: 30 minutes

Per Serving: Calories 77, Total Fat 4g, Saturated Fat 0.5g, Total Carbs 10g, Net Carbs 6g, Protein 2g, Sugar: 6g, Fiber: 4g, Sodium: 142mg, Potassium: 363mg, Phosphorus: 48mg

Ingredients:

- 2 cups diced carrots
- 1 cup peas
- 2 tablespoons olive oil
- 2 28-ounce cans of diced tomatoes
- 4 tablespoons fresh basil
- 6 cups of water
- 4 cloves of garlic
- 2 large onions, chopped
- 64 ounces vegetable broth
- 2 cups broccoli florets
- Salt and pepper to taste

Procedure:

1. First, press the Sauté button on the Instant Pot and heat the oil.
2. Sauté the garlic and onion until fragrant for 30 seconds or until fragrant.
3. Then stir in the carrots and peas and stir for 2 minutes.

4. Add in the rest of the ingredients and give a good stir.
5. Now close the lid and set the vent to the Sealing position.
6. Press the Broth/Soup button and cook on high.
7. Adjust the cooking time to 20 minutes.
8. After that, ao natural pressure release.

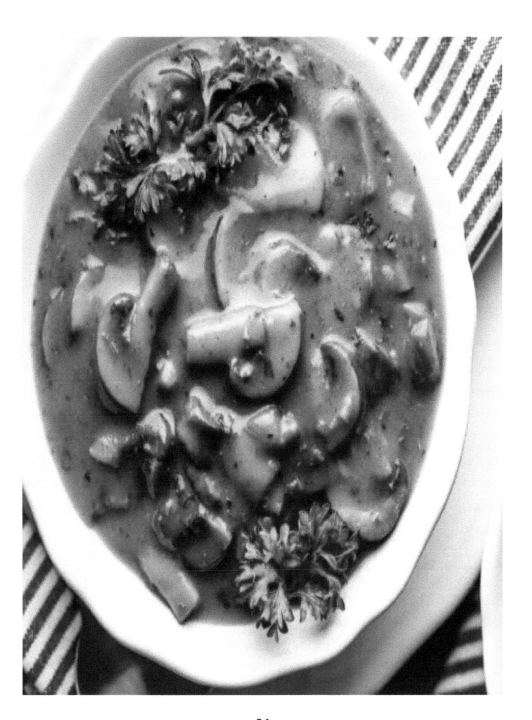

Mushroom Soup Vegetarian

Servings: 8

Preparation Time: 12 minutes

Per Serving: Calories 240, Total Fat 7g, Saturated Fat 5g, Total Carbs 35g, Net Carbs 28g, Protein 12g, Sugar: 13g, Fiber: 7g, Sodium: 440mg, Potassium: 930mg, Phosphorus: 310mg

Ingredients:

- Salt to taste
- 1 cup of water
- 1 teaspoon ground cumin
- 3 cups of coconut milk
- 16 ounces sliced cremini mushrooms
- 2 cups frozen peas
- 2 onions, chopped
- 2 28-ounce diced tomatoes
- 2 tablespoons grated ginger
- 2 tablespoons sugar
- 1 cup cilantro, chopped

Procedure:

1. Take the Instant Pot, combine the mushrooms, peas, onions, tomatoes, water, cumin, coconut milk, and ginger.
2. After that, season with salt and sugar.

3. Then close the lid and set the vent to the Sealing position.
4. Press the Pressure Cook or Manual button and adjust the cooking time to 6 minutes.
5. Do natural pressure release.
6. Once the lid is open, stir in the cilantro before serving.

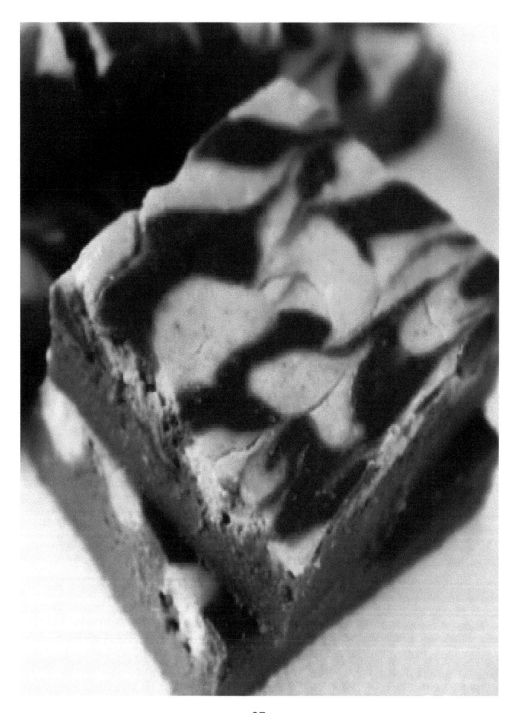

Easy Pumpkin Brownie

Servings: 8

Preparation Time: 20 minutes

Ingredients:

- 1 cup pumpkin puree
- 4 tbsps pure date sugar
- 6 oz. dairy-free dark chocolate
- 2 tbsps coconut oil
- 1/4 cup whole-wheat flour
- 1 tsp baking powder

Procedure:

1. Firstly, microwave chocolate and coconut oil for 90 seconds.
2. Mix in pumpkin purée and sugar.
3. Then stir in flour, baking powder, and a pinch of salt. Pour the batter into ramekins.
4. Arrange on a baking dish and pour in 2 cups of water.
5. Now bake for 20 minutes at 360 F.
6. Finally, let cool for a few minutes. Serve topped with raspberries.

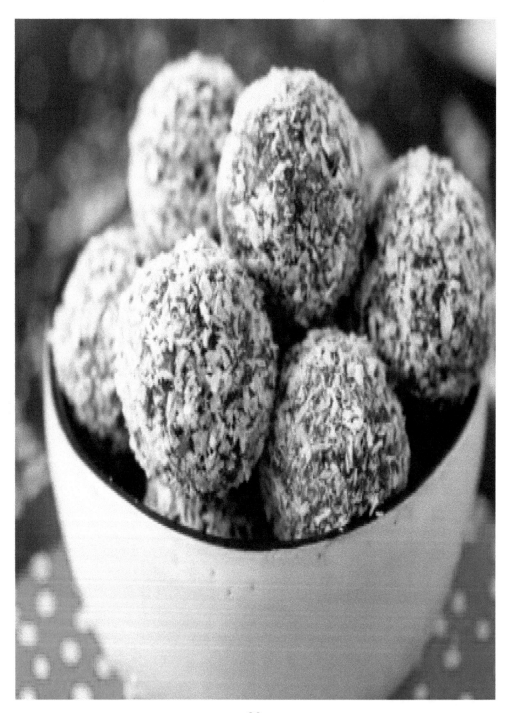

Walnut Coconut Date Truffles

Servings: 8

Preparation Time: 15 minutes

Ingredients:

- ½ cup shredded coconut
- ¼ cup pure maple syrup
- 1 cup pitted dates
- 1 cup walnuts
- ½ cup sweetened cocoa powder, plus extra for coating
- 1 tsp vanilla extract
- ¼ tsp salt

Procedure:

1. First, blend the dates, walnuts, cocoa powder, maple syrup, vanilla extract, and salt in a food processor until smooth.
2. Let chill in the fridge for 1 hour.
3. Then shape the mixture into balls and roll up the truffles in cocoa powder.
4. Now serve chilled.

Mango, Pumpkin & Lemon Cake

Servings: 16

Preparation Time: 60 minutes

Ingredients:

- 1 tsp baking powder
- 1/2 cup canola oil
- 4 tsps grated lemon zest
- 4 tbsps water
- 3 cups whole-grain flour
- 1 1/2 cup pure date sugar
- 1/2 cup yellow cornmeal
- 2 tsps baking soda
- 1 tsp salt
- 2 mangoes, chopped
- 1 tsp ground cinnamon
- 1 tsp ground allspice
- 1 tsp ground ginger
- 2 cups pumpkin puree

Procedure:

1. Firstly, preheat the oven to 360 F.
2. Secondly, take a bowl, mix flour, sugar, cornmeal, baking soda, salt, baking powder, cinnamon, allspice, and ginger.
3. Take another bowl, whisk pumpkin puree, oil, lemon zest, and water until blend.

4. Add in the mango. Pour the flour mixture into the pumpkin mixture and toss to coat.
5. Then pour the batter into a greased baking pan and bake for 45-50 minutes.
6. Let cool before slicing.

Dried Apricots & Jasmine Rice Pudding

Servings: 8

Preparation Time: 20 minutes

Per Serving: Calories: 300; Fat: 2.2g; Carbs: 63.6g; Protein: 5.6g

Ingredients:

- 2 cups water
- 2 cups almond milk
- 2 cups jasmine rice, rinsed
- 1 cup dried apricots, chopped
- ½ teaspoon cinnamon powder
- 2 teaspoons vanilla extract
- 1 cup brown sugar
- A pinch of salt
- A pinch of grated nutmeg

Procedure:

1. First, add the rice and water to a saucepan.
2. Cover the saucepan and bring the water to a boil.
3. Then turn the heat to low; let it simmer for another 10 minutes until all the water is absorbed.
4. Then, add in the remaining ingredients and stir to combine.
5. Now let it simmer for 10 minutes more or until the pudding has thickened.

Energy Bars for Everyday

Servings: 8

Preparation Time: 35 minutes

Per Serving: Calories: 285; Fat: 17.1g; Carbs: 30g; Protein: 5.1g

Ingredients:

- 4 cups old-fashioned oats
- 1 cup almonds, slivered
- 1 cup walnuts, chopped
- 1/2 cup vegan butter
- 1/2 cup brown sugar
- 4 tablespoons agave syrup
- 1 cup dried currants
- 1 cup pepitas

Procedure:

1. First, begin by preheating your oven to 320 degrees F.
2. Line a baking pan with parchment paper or a Silpat mat.
3. Then thoroughly combine all the ingredients until everything is well incorporated.
4. Spread the mixture onto the prepared baking pan using a wide spatula.
5. Now bake for about 33 minutes or until golden brown.
6. Finally, cut into bars using a sharp knife and enjoy!

Raw Coconut Ice Cream

Servings: 4

Preparation Time: 10 minutes

Per Serving: Calories: 388; Fat: 7.7g; Carbs: 82g; Protein: 4.8g

Ingredients:

- 8 tablespoons coconut milk
- 12 fresh dates, pitted
- 1/2 teaspoon pure coconut extract
- 8 over-ripe bananas, frozen
- 1 teaspoon pure vanilla extract
- 1 cup coconut flakes

Procedure:

1. First, place all the ingredients in the bowl of your food processor or high-speed blender.
2. Blitz the ingredients until creamy or until your desired consistency is achieved.
3. Then serve immediately or store in your freezer.

BREAKFAST

Apply Honey Toast

Servings: 8

Preparation Time: 5 minutes

Per Serving: Calories: 212 Cal Fat: 7 g Carbs: 35 g Protein: 4 g Fiber: 5.5 g

Ingredients:

- 1 of a small apple, cored, sliced
- 4 tablespoons hummus
- 1/4 teaspoon cinnamon
- 2 slices of whole-grain bread, toasted
- 2 tablespoons honey

Procedure:

1. First, spread hummus on one side of the toast, top with apple slices, and then drizzle with honey.
2. Now, sprinkle cinnamon on it and then serve straight away.

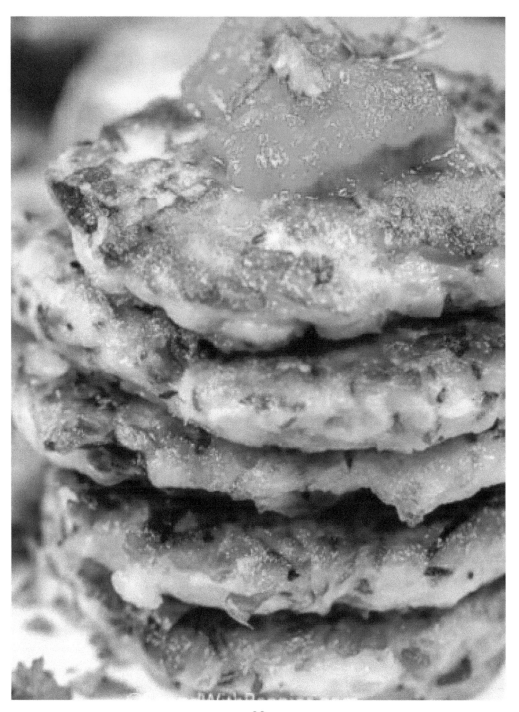

Homemade Zucchini Pancakes

Servings: 8

Preparation Time: 25 minutes

Per Serving: Calories 65, Total Fat 4.7g, Saturated Fat 0.9g, Cholesterol 41mg, Sodium 97mg, Total Carbohydrate 4.1g, Dietary Fiber 0.8g, Total Sugars 1.4g, Protein 2.3g, Calcium 16mg, Iron 1mg, Potassium 175mg, Phosphorus 24mg

Ingredients:

- 2 teaspoons herb seasoning
- 2 eggs
- 2 tablespoons olive oil
- 4 cups zucchini
- 1/2 cup onion
- 2 tablespoons all-purpose white flour
- 1/4 teaspoon salt

Procedure:

1. First, grate onion and zucchini into a bowl and stir to combine.
2. Place the zucchini mixture on a clean kitchen towel.
3. Then twist and squeeze out as much liquid as possible.
4. Return to the bowl.
5. Now mix flour, salt, and herb seasoning in a small bowl.

6. After that, add egg and mix; stir into zucchini and onion mixture. Form 4 patties.
7. Heat oil over high heat in a large nonstick frying pan.
8. Then lower heat to medium and place zucchini patties into the pan.
9. Sauté until brown, turning once.

Spinach & Mushroom Crepes

Servings: 8

Preparation Time: 1 ½ hour

Per Serving: Calories: 680, Total Fat: 71.8g, Saturated Fat:20.9g, Total Carbs:10g, Dietary Fiber:7g, Sugar:2g, Protein:3g, Sodium:525mg

Ingredients:

For the crepes:

- 3 cups of soy milk
- 3 1/2 cups rolled oats
- 2 tbsps almond butter
- 1 tsp nutmeg
- 4 tbsps egg replacement
- 2 tsps pink Himalayan salt
- 4 tbsps olive oil

For the filling:

- 2 lbs button mushrooms
- 2 tbsps fresh rosemary, finely chopped
- 2 garlic cloves, crushed
- 4 tbsps olive oil
- 20 oz. fresh spinach, finely chopped
- 8 oz. crumbled tofu
- 2 tbsps chia seeds

Procedure:

1. First, prepare the crepes.
2. Combine all dry ingredients in a large bowl.
3. Add milk, butter, nutmeg, olive oil, and egg replacement.
4. Mix well with a hand mixer at high speed.
5. Transfer to a food processor and process until completely smooth.
6. Grease a large nonstick pancake pan with some oil.
7. Pour 1 cup of the mixture into the pan and cook for one minute on each side.
8. Plug your instant pot and press the 'Sauté' button.
9. Grease the stainless steel insert with some oil and add mushrooms.
10. Cook for 5 minutes, stirring constantly.
11. Now add spinach, tofu, rosemary, and garlic. Continue to cook for another 5 minutes.
12. Remove the mixture from the pot and stir in chia seeds. Let it sit for 10 minutes.
13. Meanwhile, grease a small baking pan with some oil and line it with parchment paper.
14. Divide the mushroom mixture between crepes and roll-up.
15. Gently transfer to a prepared baking pan.
16. Wrap the pan with aluminum foil and set it aside.
17. Pour 1 cup of water into your instant pot and set the steam rack. Put the pan on top and seal the lid.

18. Press the 'Manual' button and set the timer for 10 minutes.
19. When done, release the pressure naturally, and open the lid.
20. Optionally, sprinkle with some dried oregano before serving.

Perfect Berry Quinoa Bowl

Servings: 8

Preparation Time: 5 minutes

Ingredients:

- 4 cups berries
- 1 cup chopped raw hazelnuts
- 2 1/2 cups unsweetened almond milk
- 4 bananas, sliced
- 1/2 cup agave syrup
- 6 cups cooked quinoa

Procedure:

1. Take a large bowl, combine the quinoa, milk, banana, raspberries, blueberries, and hazelnuts.
2. Then divide between serving bowls and top with agave syrup to serve.

Breakfast Gallete

Servings: 10

Preparation Time: 40 minutes

Per Serving: Calories: 208; Fat: 7.7g; Carbs: 27.7g; Protein: 4.8g

Ingredients:

- 1/2 teaspoon ground allspice
- 2 cups water
- 1 cup rice milk
- 2 teaspoons brown sugar
- 2 cups all-purpose flour
- 1 cup oat flour
- 2 teaspoons baking powder
- 2 teaspoons baking soda
- 1 teaspoon kosher salt
- 4 tablespoons olive oil

Procedure:

1. First, mix the flour, baking powder, baking soda, salt, sugar, and ground allspice using an electric mixer.
2. Gradually pour in the water, milk, and oil and continue mixing until everything is well incorporated.
3. Then heat a lightly greased griddle over medium-high heat.

4. Ladle 1/4 of the batter into the preheated griddle and cook until your galette is golden and crisp.
5. Repeat with the remaining batter.
6. Serve your galette with homemade jelly, if desired. Bon appétit!

Morning Chocolate Crunch

Servings: 5

Preparation Time: 35 minutes

Per Serving: Calories: 372; Fat: 19.9g; Carbs: 43.7g; Protein: 8.2g

Ingredients:

- 1/4 cup chocolate chunks
- 1/2 cup rolled oats
- 1/4 cup pecans, chopped
- ¼ cup rye flakes
- 1/4 cup buckwheat flakes
- 1/2 teaspoon vanilla paste
- 1/4 teaspoon pumpkin spice mix
- 1/8 cup coconut oil, softened
- 1/4 cup hazelnuts, chopped
- 1/2 cup coconut, shredded
- 1/4 cup date syrup

Procedure:

1. First of all, start by preheating your oven to 330 degrees F. Line a baking sheet with parchment paper or a Silpat mat.
2. Take a mixing bowl, thoroughly combine all the ingredients, except for the chocolate chunks.
3. Then, spread the cereal mixture onto the prepared baking sheet.

4. Bake for about 33 minutes or until crunchy.
5. Fold the chocolate chunks into the warm cereal mixture.
6. Now allow it to cool fully before breaking up into clumps.
7. Finally, serve with plant-based milk of choice.

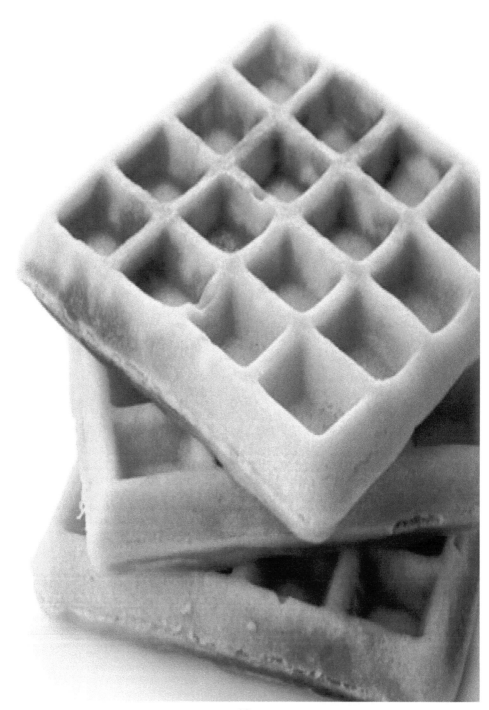

Breakfast Wafers

Servings: 8

Preparation Time: 30 minutes

Per Serving: : Calories: 288; Fat: 11.1g; Carbs: 45.3g; Protein: 4.4g

Ingredients:

- 1 cup instant oats
- 2 teaspoons baking powder
- 1 teaspoon baking soda
- 2 1/2 cups rice flour
- 1/2 cup tapioca flour
- 1 cup potato starch
- 3 cups oat milk
- 2 teaspoons apple cider vinegar
- 1/2 cup coconut oil, softened
- 1/2 cup maple syrup
- 2 pinches sea salt
- 1 teaspoon vanilla essence
- 1 teaspoon cinnamon

Procedure:

1. Preheat a waffle iron according to the manufacturer's instructions.
2. Take a mixing bowl, thoroughly combine the flour, potato starch, instant oats, baking powder, baking soda, salt, vanilla, and cinnamon.

3. Then gradually add in the milk, whisking continuously to avoid lumps.
4. Add in the apple cider vinegar, coconut oil, and maple syrup. Whisk again to combine well.
5. Now beat until everything is well blended.
6. Ladle 1/2 cup of the batter into the preheated iron and cook according to manufacturer instructions until your wafers are golden.
7. After that, repeat with the remaining batter.
8. Serve with toppings of choice.

Ukrainian Blinis

Servings: 12

Preparation Time: 1 hour

Per Serving: Calories: 138; Fat: 5.7g; Carbs: 17.9g; Protein: 3.4g

Ingredients:

- 2 pinches of salt
- 2 pinches of grated nutmeg
- 4 tablespoons olive oil
- 2 teaspoons yeast
- 2 teaspoons brown sugar
- 1 1/2 cups oat milk
- 1 cups all-purpose flour
- 2 pinches of ground cloves

Procedure:

1. Place the yeast, sugar, and 2 tablespoons of the lukewarm milk in a small mixing bowl; whisk to combine and let it dissolve and ferment for about 10 minutes.
2. Take a mixing bowl, combine the flour with the salt, nutmeg, and cloves; add in the yeast mixture and stir to combine well.
3. Then gradually pour in the milk and stir until everything is well incorporated.

4. Let the batter sit for about 30 minutes in a warm place.
5. Heat a small amount of the oil in a nonstick skillet over a moderate flame.
6. Drop the batter, 1/4 cup at a time, onto the preheated skillet. Fry until bubbles form or about 2 minutes.
7. Flip your blini and continue frying until brown, about 2 minutes more. Repeat with the remaining oil and batter,
8. Serve with toppings of choice.

Old fashioned Corn Bread

Servings: 10

Preparation Time: 50 minutes

Per Serving: Calories: 388; Fat: 23.7g; Carbs: 39g; Protein: 4.7g

Ingredients:

- 2 teaspoons baking powder
- 2 teaspoons baking soda
- 3 cups plain flour
- 2 cups cornmeal
- 2 teaspoons kosher salt
- 1/2 cup sugar
- 4 tablespoons chia seeds
- 3 cups oat milk
- 1/2 cup olive oil

Procedure:

1. First, start by preheating your oven to 420 degrees F.
2. Now, spritz a baking pan with a nonstick cooking spray.
3. Then to make the chia "egg," mix 2 tablespoons of the chia seeds with 4 tablespoons of water.
4. Now stir and let it sit for about 15 minutes.

5. Take a mixing bowl, thoroughly combine the flour, cornmeal, baking powder, baking soda, salt, and sugar.
6. Then, gradually add in the chia "egg," oat milk, and olive oil, constantly whisking to avoid lumps.
7. Scrape the batter into the prepared baking pan.
8. Bake your cornbread for about 25 minutes or until a tester inserted in the middle comes out dry and clean.
9. In the end, let it stand for about 10 minutes before slicing and serving.

Morning Tangerine Banana Toast

Servings: 8

Preparation Time: 25 minutes

Ingredients:

- 2 tsps ground cinnamon
- 1/2 tsp grated nutmeg
- 8 slices bread
- 6 bananas
- 2 cups almond milk
- Zest and juice of 1 tangerine
- 2 tbsps olive oil

Procedure:

1. Blend the bananas, almond milk, tangerine juice, tangerine zest, cinnamon, and nutmeg until smooth in a food processor.
2. Spread into a baking dish. Submerge the bread slices in the mixture for 3-4 minutes.
3. Heat the oil in a skillet over medium heat.
4. Fry the bread for 5 minutes until golden brown. Serve hot.

Easy Maple Banana Oats

Servings: 8

Preparation Time: 35 minutes

Ingredients:

- 1/2 cup pumpkin seeds
- 4 tbsps maple syrup
- 6 cups water
- 2 cups steel-cut oats
- 4 bananas, mashed
- A pinch of salt

Procedure:

1. First, bring water to a boil in a pot, add in oats, and lower the heat.
2. Cook for 20-30 minutes.
3. Then put in the mashed bananas, cook for 3-5 minutes more.
4. Stir in maple syrup, pumpkin seeds, and salt.

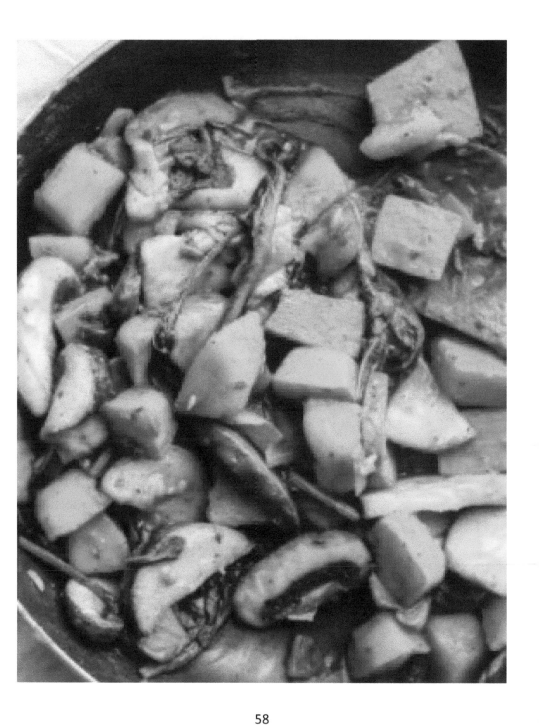

Pumpkin Stir Fry

Servings: 4

Preparation Time: 25 minutes

Ingredients:

- 4 garlic cloves, minced
- 1 tsp dried thyme
- 2 cups chopped kale
- 2 carrots, peeled and chopped
- Salt and black pepper to taste
- 2 cups pumpkin, shredded
- 2 tbsps olive oil
- 1 onion, chopped

Procedure:

1. First, heat the oil in a skillet over medium heat.
2. Sauté onion and carrot for 5 minutes.
3. Now add in garlic and thyme, cook for 30 seconds until the garlic is fragrant.
4. Place in the pumpkin and cook for 10 minutes until tender. Stir in kale, cook for 4 minutes until the kale wilts.
5. Then season with salt and pepper. Serve hot.

MAIN DISHES

Avocado & Butternut Squash Chipotle Chili

Servings: 8

Preparation Time: 40 minutes

Per Serving: Calories: 140 Cal Fat: 0.9 g Carbs: 27.1 g
Protein: 6.3 g Fiber: 6.2 g

Ingredients:

- 6 cups black beans, cooked
- 2 onions, chopped
- 4 bell peppers, chopped
- 2 small butternut squashes, cubed
- In adobo
- 2 teaspoons ground cumin
- 1/2 teaspoon ground cinnamon
- 28 oz. can diced tomatoes, including the liquid
- 4 cups vegetable broth
- 2 bay leaves
- 4 avocados, diced
- 6 corn tortillas for crispy tortilla strips
- Salt
- 8 garlic cloves, minced
- 4 tablespoons olive oil
- 2 tablespoons chili powder
- 1 tablespoon chopped chipotle pepper

Procedure:

1. First, place a stockpot over medium heat. Add oil.
2. Then add and cook onion, bell peppers, and butternut squash for about 5 minutes.
3. Reduce the heat, add garlic, chili powder, ½ tablespoon chopped chipotle peppers, cumin, and cinnamon.
4. Now cook for ½ a minute.
5. Add bay leaves, black beans, tomatoes, and their juices and broth and mix well.
6. Cook for about 1 hour. Remove bay leaf when done cooking.
7. Then slice corn tortillas into thin little strips.
8. Place a pan over medium heat and add olive oil.
9. After that, add tortilla strips and season with salt.
10. Cook until crispy for about 7 minutes.
11. Remove from the heat and place in a bowl covered with a paper towel to drain excess oil.
12. Finally, serve chili in bowls, topped with crispy tortilla chips and avocado.

Easy Chickpea Biryani

Servings: 12

Preparation Time: 1 hour

Per Serving: Calories: 140 Cal Fat: 0.9 g Carbs: 27.1 g
Protein: 6.3 g Fiber: 6.2 g

Ingredients:

- 2 tablespoons cumin
- 1 teaspoon turmeric
- 1 cup raisins
- 2 large onions, thinly sliced
- 4 cups thinly sliced veggies (bell pepper, zucchini, and carrots)
- 8 cups veggie stock
- 4 cups basmati rice, rinsed
- 2 cans chickpeas, drained, rinsed
- 6 garlic cloves, chopped
- 2 tablespoons ginger, chopped
- 4 tablespoons olive oil
- 2 bays leafs
- 2 tablespoons coriander
- 2 teaspoons chili powder
- 2 teaspoons cinnamon
- 1 teaspoon cardamom
- Salt

Procedure:

1. First, place a large skillet over medium-high heat. Add oil.
2. Sauté onions for about 5 minutes.
3. Reduce the heat to medium, add vegetables, garlic, and ginger.
4. Then cook for 5 minutes. Scoop 1 cup of this mixture and set aside.
5. Add spices, bay leaf, and rice. Stir for about 1 minute.
6. Now add stock and salt to taste.
7. After that, add chickpeas, raisins, and 1 cup of vegetables.
8. Bring the mixture to a simmer over high heat.
9. Lower the heat, cover tightly and let it simmer for ½ an hour.
10. In conclusion, remove from the heat when rice is done.

Homemade Chinese Eggplant

Servings: 1 ½ hour

Preparation Time: 8

Per Serving: Calories:680, Total Fat:71.8g, Saturated Fat:20.9g, Total Carbs:10g, Dietary Fiber:7g, Sugar:2g, Protein:3g, Sodium:525mg

Ingredients:

- 8 tablespoons peanut oil
- 3 lbs. eggplants, chopped
- 4 cups of water
- 4 teaspoons ginger, minced
- 20 dried red chilies
- Salt
- 4 tablespoons cornstarch
- 8 cloves garlic, chopped

For the Szechuan sauce:

- 6 tablespoons coconut sugar
- 1 teaspoon five-spice
- 2 teaspoons Szechuan peppercorns
- 1/2 cup of soy sauce
- 2 tablespoons garlic chili paste
- 2 tablespoons sesame oil
- 2 tablespoons rice vinegar
- 2 tablespoons Chinese cooking wine

Procedure:

1. First, place chopped eggplants in a shallow bowl.
2. Add water and 4 teaspoons of salt.
3. Stir cover and let it sit for about 15 minutes.
4. Then meanwhile, place a small pan over medium heat.
5. Toast the Szechuan peppercorns for about 2 minutes and crush them.
6. Now add crushed peppercorns to a medium bowl, add soy, chili paste, sesame oil, rice vinegar, Chinese cooking vinegar, coconut sugar, and five spices.
7. Drain excess liquid from the eggplants and toss in the corn starch.
8. After that, place a large skillet over medium heat, add eggplants and cook them until golden. Set aside.
9. Add 1 tablespoon of oil to the skillet placed over medium heat. Cook garlic and ginger for 2 minutes.
10. Then add dried chilies and cook for 1 minute.
11. Add the Szechuan sauce and bring the mixture to a simmer in 20 seconds.
12. Finally, add back eggplants and cook for about 60 seconds.

Bok Choy & Black Pepper Tofu

Servings: 4

Preparation Time: 1 hour

Per Serving: Calories: 140 Cal Fat: 0.9 g Carbs: 27.1 g Protein: 6.3 g Fiber: 6.2 g

Ingredients:

- 24 oz. firm tofu, cubed
- 2 teaspoon freshly cracked peppercorns
- 2 shallot, sliced
- 8 cloves of garlic, chopped
- 1 cup cornstarch for dredging
- 4 tablespoons coconut oil
- 12 oz. baby bok choy, sliced into 4 slices

For the black pepper sauce:

- 4 tablespoons soy sauce
- 4 tablespoons Chinese cooking wine
- 1 teaspoon freshly cracked peppercorns
- 2 teaspoons chili paste
- 4 tablespoons water
- 2 teaspoons brown sugar

Procedure:

1. Take a small bowl, combine wok sauce ingredients and mix well until sugar dissolves and set aside.

2. Place cornstarch in a shallow bowl and dredge tofu in the cornstarch, and set aside.
3. Then place a large skillet over medium heat.
4. Heat 1 tablespoon coconut oil.
5. Add peppercorns and toast for about 1 minute.
6. Now add tofu and cook on all sides for about 6 minutes. Set tofu aside.
7. After that, add the remaining coconut oil. Add shallots, garlic, and bok choy.
8. Cook for 8 minutes.
9. Add back the tofu and cook for less than a minute.

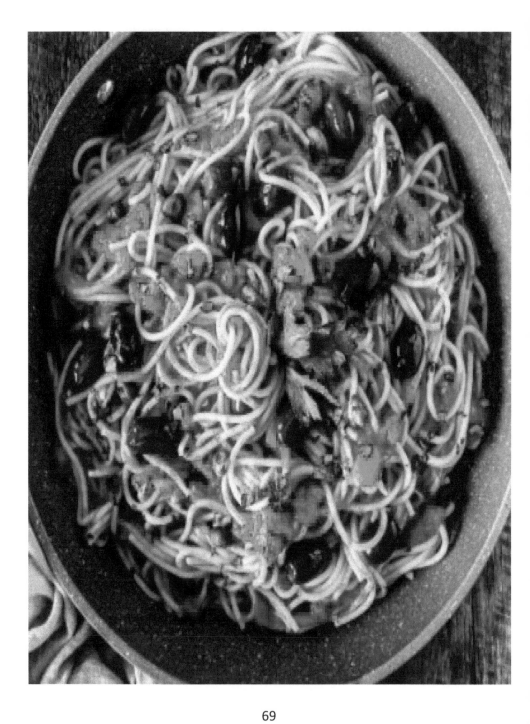

Alla Puttanesca Spaghetti

Servings: 8

Preparation Time: 1 hour

Per Serving: Calories: 140 Cal Fat: 0.9 g Carbs: 27.1 g
Protein: 6.3 g Fiber: 6.2 g

Ingredients:

For the Puttanesca sauce:

- 56 oz. can chunky tomato sauce
- 1/2 teaspoon red pepper flakes
- 2 tablespoons caper brine
- 6 cloves garlic, minced
- 2 tablespoons olive oil
- 1 cup parsley leaves, chopped and divided
- salt and pepper
- 1/2 cup chopped Kalamata olives
- 1/2 cup capers
- 2 tablespoons Kalamata olive brine

For the pasta:

- 12 oz. zucchini noodles
- 16 oz. whole-grain spaghetti

Procedure:

1. Firstly, place a medium skillet over medium heat.

2. Add tomato sauce, olives, capers, olive brine, caper brine, garlic, and red pepper flakes.
3. Then bring the mixture to a boil, reduce the heat, and let it simmer for 20 minutes.
4. Remove from the heat and set aside.
5. Now place a pot over medium heat. Add water, salt, spaghetti, and cook as directed on the package. When done, drain excess water.
6. Pour the sauce over pasta and mix well.
7. After that, add zucchini noodles before serving.

Grilled Zucchini & Kale Pizza

Servings: 8

Preparation Time: 30 minutes

Ingredients:

- 1/2 cup capers
- 2 tsps salt
- 4 large zucchinis, sliced
- 1 cup chopped kale
- 2 tsps oregano
- 2 pinches sugar
- 1 cup grated plant Parmesan cheese
- 7 cups whole-wheat flour
- 2 tsps yeast
- 6 tbsps olive oil
- 2 cups marinara sauce

Procedure:

1. First of all, preheat the oven to 350 F and lightly grease a pizza pan with cooking spray. In a bowl, mix flour, nutritional yeast, salt, sugar, olive oil, and 1 cup of warm water until smooth dough forms.
2. Allow rising for an hour or until the dough doubles in size.
3. Then spread the dough on the pizza pan and apply marinara sauce and oregano on top.

4. Heat a grill pan, season the zucchinis with salt, black pepper, and cook in the pan until slightly charred on both sides.
5. Now sit the zucchini on the pizza crust and top with kale, capers, and plant-based Parmesan cheese. Bake for 20 minutes.
6. Finally, cool for 5 minutes, slice, and serve.

Tofu Burger

Servings: 8

Preparation Time: 20 minutes

Ingredients:

- 2 tbsps toasted almond flour
- 2 tbsps flax seed powder
- 1/4 lb. crumbled tofu
- 1/2 tsp curry powder
- 6 tbsps whole-grain breadcrumbs
- 8 whole-wheat burger buns, halved
- 2 tbsps quick-cooking oats
- 1 tsp garlic powder
- 1 tsp onion powder

Procedure:

1. Take a small bowl, mix the flax seed powder with 6 tbsps of water and allow thickening for 5 minutes to make the vegan "flax egg.
2. Then set aside. In a bowl, mix tofu, oats, almond flour, garlic powder, onion powder, salt, pepper, and curry powder.
3. Mold 4 patties out of the mixture and brush both sides with the vegan "flax egg.
4. Now pour the breadcrumbs onto a plate and coat the cakes in the crumbs until well covered.

5. Heat a pan over medium heat and grease with cooking spray.
6. Then cook the patties on both sides for 10 minutes.
7. Place each patty between each burger bun and top with the guacamole. Serve immediately.

Bean Gyros

Servings: 12

Preparation Time: 60 minutes

Ingredients:

- 2 cups hummus
- 2 cups arugula, chopped
- 1/2 cup fresh parsley, chopped
- 4 tbsps Kalamata olives, chopped
- 2 tbsps tahini
- 2 (28-oz) cans of white beans
- 4 scallions, minced
- 2 cucumbers, chopped
- 1/2 cup chopped avocado
- 1/2 tsp paprika
- 8 tsps olive oil
- 12 whole-grain wraps, warm
- 2 tbsps lemon juice
- 1 tsp ground cumin
- 4 tomatoes, chopped

Procedure:

1. Take a blender, place the white beans, scallions, parsley, and olives. Pulse until finely chopped. In a bowl, beat the tahini with lemon juice.
2. Add in cumin, paprika, and salt.

3. Then transfer into beans mixture and mix well to combine. Shape the mixture into balls; flatten to make 6 patties.
4. Take a skillet over medium heat, warm the oil and cook the patties for 8-10 minutes on both sides; reserve.
5. Spread each wrap with hummus and top with patties, tomatoes, cucumber, and avocado.
6. Finally, roll the wraps up to serve.

Asparagus & Mushroom with Mashed Potatoes

Servings: 8

Preparation Time: 60 minutes

Ingredients:

- 6 tsp coconut oil
- 4 tbsps nutritional yeast
- 4 tsps olive oil
- 1 cup non-dairy milk
- 4 tbsps nutritional yeast
- 10 large portobello mushrooms, stems removed
- 12 potatoes, chopped
- 8 garlic cloves, minced
- 14 cups asparagus, chopped
- Sea salt to taste

Procedure:

1. First, place the chopped potatoes in a pot and cover them with salted water.
2. Cook for 20 minutes.
3. Then heat oil in a skillet and sauté garlic for 1 minute.
4. Once the potatoes are ready, drain them and reserve the water.
5. Now transfer to a bowl and mash them with some hot water, garlic, milk, yeast, and salt.

6. Then preheat your grill to medium. Grease the mushrooms with cooking spray and season with salt.
7. Arrange the mushrooms face down and grill for 10 minutes.
8. After, grill the asparagus for about 10 minutes, turning often. Arrange the veggies in a serving platter.
9. Finally, add in the potato mash and serve.

Simple Black Bean Stuffed Avocado

Servings: 12

Preparation Time: 10 minutes

Per Serving: Calories: 247; Fat: 18.9g; Carbs: 19.3g;
Protein: 5.2g

Ingredients:

- 2 teaspoons red pepper flakes
- 4 tablespoons fresh mint, roughly chopped
- 4 tablespoons balsamic glaze reduction to drizzle
- 6 tablespoons tahini
- 2 garlic cloves, minced
- 6 avocados, seeded and cut into halves
- 2 lemons, freshly squeezed
- 2 cups cherry tomatoes, quartered
- 12 tablespoons black beans, mashed
- Sea salt and ground black pepper, to taste

Procedure:

1. Firstly, place your avocados on a serving platter.
2. Then drizzle the lemon juice over each avocado.
3. Take a mixing bowl, stir the remaining ingredients for the stuffing until well incorporated.
4. Fill the avocados with the prepared mixture and serve immediately. Bon appétit!

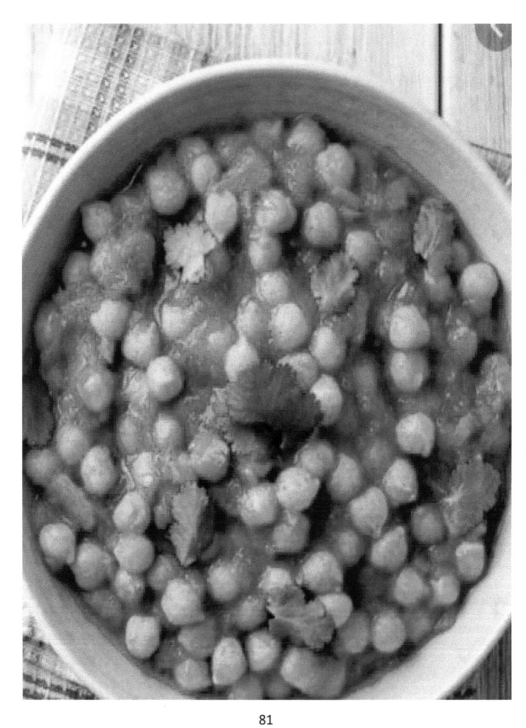

Chickpea Curry

Servings: 8

Preparation Time: 15 minutes

Per Serving: Calories: 505; Fat: 37.7g; Carbs: 37.2g; Protein: 11.7g

Ingredients:

- 2 teaspoons fresh ginger, minced
- 4 garlic cloves, peeled
- 2 teaspoons curry powder
- 28 ounces canned chickpeas, drained
- 2 onions, diced
- 2 Thai chili peppers
- 4 ripe tomatoes, diced
- 1 cup vegetable broth
- 2 (27-ounce) cans coconut milk, unsweetened
- 2 teaspoons cumin seeds
- 1 teaspoon mustard seeds
- 2 bays leafs
- 2 limes, freshly squeezed
- 6 tablespoons coconut oil
- Sea salt and ground black pepper, to taste
- 2 tablespoons garam masala

Procedure:

1. Take your blender or food processor, blend the onion, chili pepper, tomatoes, ginger, garlic, cumin, mustard, and bay leaf into a paste.
2. Take a saucepan, heat the coconut oil over medium heat. Once hot, cook the prepared paste for about 2 minutes or until aromatic.
3. Then add in the salt, pepper, garam masala, curry powder canned, chickpeas, vegetable broth, and coconut milk.
4. Turn the heat to a simmer.
5. Now continue to simmer for 8 minutes more or until cooked through.
6. Remove from the heat. Drizzle fresh lime juice over the top of each serving.

One-Pot Chili with Tofu

Servings: 8

Preparation Time: 1 hour 30 minutes

Per Serving: Calories: 605; Fat: 20.1g; Carbs: 74g; Protein: 38.3g

Ingredients:

- 6 tablespoons olive oil
- 2 large onions, diced
- 2 tablespoons red chili powder
- 2 tablespoons brown sugar
- Sea salt and cayenne pepper, to taste
- 24 ounces silken tofu, cubed
- 1 ½ pounds cannellini beans, soaked overnight and drained
- 2 cups turnip, chopped
- 2 carrots, chopped
- 2 bell peppers, sliced
- 2 sweet potatoes, chopped
- 6 cloves garlic, minced
- 4 ripe tomatoes, pureed
- 6 tablespoons tomato paste
- 4 cups vegetable broth
- 4 bay leaves

Procedure:

1. First, cover the soaked beans with a fresh change of cold water and bring them to a boil.
2. Let it boil for about 10 minutes.
3. Then turn the heat to a simmer and continue to cook for 50 to 55 minutes or until tender.
4. Take a heavy-bottomed pot, heat the olive oil over medium heat.
5. Once hot, sauté the onion, turnip, carrot, bell pepper, and sweet potato.
6. Sauté the garlic for about 1 minute or so.
7. Now add in the tomatoes, tomato paste, vegetable broth, bay leaves, red chili powder, brown sugar, salt, cayenne pepper, and cooked beans.
8. Let it simmer, stirring periodically, for 25 to 30 minutes or until cooked through.
9. Finally, serve garnished with silken tofu.

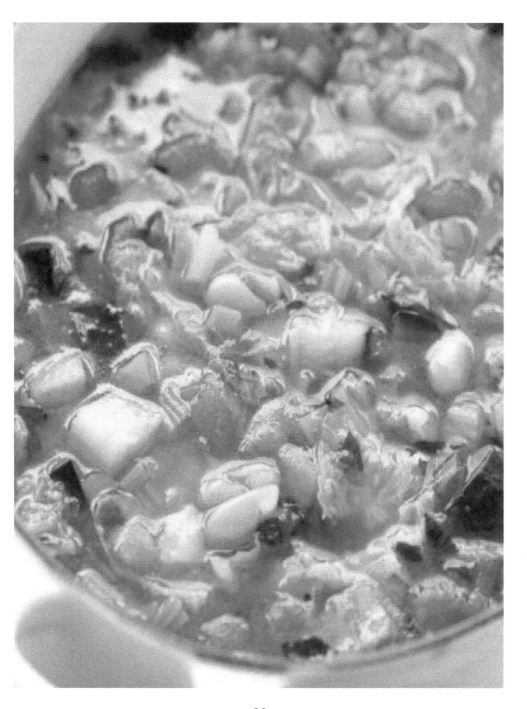

Italian Minestrone

Servings: 10

Preparation Time: 30 minutes

Per Serving: Calories: 305; Fat: 8.6g; Carbs: 45.1g; Protein: 14.2g

Ingredients:

- 8 cloves garlic, minced
- 2 cups elbow pasta
- 10 cups vegetable broth
- 4 tablespoons olive oil
- 2 large onions, diced
- 2 large zucchinis, diced
- 2 (56-ounce) cans tomatoes, crushed
- 2 tablespoons fresh oregano leaves, chopped
- 4 carrots, sliced
- 2 (30-ounce) cans of white beans, drained
- 2 tablespoons fresh basil leaves, chopped
- 2 tablespoons fresh Italian parsley, chopped

Procedure:

1. In a Dutch oven, heat the olive oil until sizzling.
2. Now, sauté the onion and carrots until they've softened.

3. Then add in the garlic, uncooked pasta, and broth; let it simmer for about 15 minutes.
4. Stir in the beans, zucchini, tomatoes, and herbs. Continue to cook, covered, for about 10 minutes until everything is thoroughly cooked.
5. Garnish with some extra herbs, if desired.

SIDE DISHES

BBQ Baked Beans

Servings: 4

Preparation Time: 55 minutes

Per Serving: Calories 510, Total Fat 1.4g, Saturated Fat 0.3g, Cholesterol 0mg, Sodium 661mg, Total Carbohydrate 118.1g, Dietary Fiber 14.2g, Total Sugars 82.7g, Protein 12.9g

Ingredients:

- 2 small onions, finely chopped
- 1/2 cup lemon juice
- 1 cup honey
- Enough water
- 1/2 red or green bell pepper, cored, seeded, and finely chopped
- 1/2 cup barbecue sauce
- 1 cup dry navy beans
- 4 cups of water
- 1/2 teaspoon salt
- 1 teaspoon mustard

Procedure:

1. Firstly, add navy beans, water, and salt into Instant Pot.
2. Secondly, cook on Manual (High Pressure) for 25 minutes.
3. Allow the pressure to naturally release.

4. After that, remove the lid and pour beans into a colander/strainer. Rinse with cold water. Set aside.
5. Set Instant Pot to Sauté setting.
6. Then add bell pepper and onions and cook until tender.
7. Turn IP off. Add barbecue sauce, mustard, lemon juice to the Instant pot and stir well to combine.
8. Now add honey, water, and beans and stir to combine.
9. Secure IP lid, close steam valve, and cook on Manual (High pressure) for 15 minutes.
10. Allow the pressure to naturally release.
11. In the end, carefully open the lid and gently stir the mixture to combine.

Mint Black Beans

Servings: 4

Preparation Time: 55 minutes

Per Serving: Calories 277, Total Fat 8.1g, Saturated Fat 6.1g, Cholesterol 0mg, Sodium 646mg, Total Carbohydrate 41.3g, Dietary Fiber 11. 3g, Total Sugars 6g, Protein 13g

Ingredients:

- 1 cup of dried black beans
- 1/2 teaspoon coriander powder
- 1/4 teaspoon dried basil
- 2 bay leaves
- 4 cups vegetable stock
- 1 cup halved cherry tomatoes
- 1/2 medium jalapeno pepper, seeded and finely chopped
- 2 teaspoons garlic powder
- 1 teaspoon salt
- 1 teaspoon cumin seed
- 1 cup chopped mint leaves
- 2 tablespoons coconut oil
- 1 cup chopped onions
- 1 cup chopped red bell pepper

Procedure:

1. First, set an Instant Pot to Sauté. Allow to heat for 3 minutes.

2. Add coconut oil, onions, red bell peppers, jalapeno pepper, garlic powder, salt, cumin seed, coriander powder, and basil.
3. Then cook, often stirring for about 5 minutes.
4. Add bay leaves, stock, and black beans.
5. Now stir to blend. Cover Instant Pot, and fasten the lid.
6. Lock and seal steam valve.
7. Set to High Pressure for 30 minutes.
8. After that, when the cooking time has ended, allow Instant Pot to naturally release pressure for 20 minutes.
9. Uncover and turn off Instant Pot.
10. To serve, spoon beans and cooking liquid into bowls and top evenly with cherry tomatoes and mint leaves.

Chicago Vegetable Stew

Servings: 8

Preparation Time: 35 minutes

Ingredients:

- 1/2 cup fresh basil
- ½ cup chopped fresh parsley
- 3 cups vegetable broth
- 4 tbsps olive oils
- 6 shallots, chopped
- 2 carrots, sliced
- 1 cup dry white wine
- 6 new potatoes, cubed
- 2 red bell peppers, chopped
- 2 cups green beans
- 4 zucchinis, sliced
- 2 yellow summer squashes, sliced
- 2 lbs plum tomatoes, chopped
- 4 Salt and black pepper to taste
- 6 cups fresh corn kernels

Procedure:

1. First, heat oil in a pot over medium heat.
2. Place shallots and carrot and cook for 5 minutes.
3. Then pour in white wine, potatoes, bell pepper, and broth.

4. Bring to a boil, lower the heat, and simmer for 5 minutes.
5. Now stir in zucchini, yellow squash, and tomatoes. Sprinkle with salt and pepper. Simmer for 20 more minutes.
6. Put in corn, green peas, basil, and parsley.
7. Simmer an additional 5 minutes and serve hot.

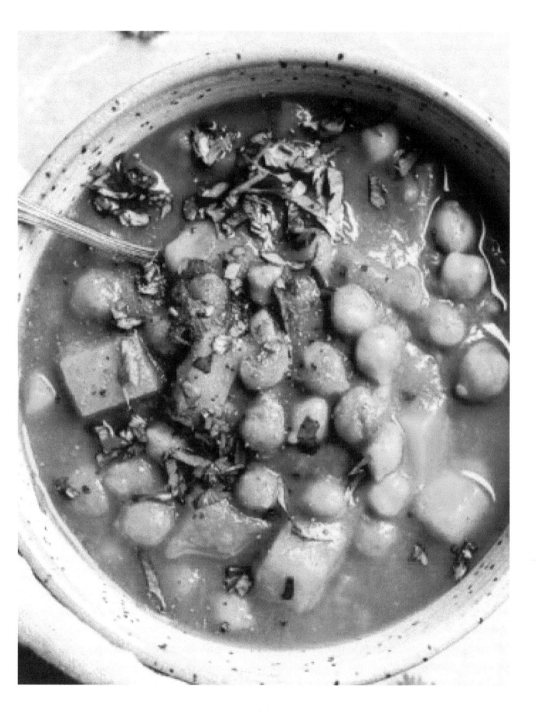

Moroccan Bean Stew

Servings: 8

Preparation Time: 40 minutes

Ingredients:

- Salt and black pepper to taste
- 6 cups eggplants, chopped
- 1/2 cup chopped roasted peanuts
- 6 garlic cloves, minced
- 2 tsps grated fresh ginger
- 1 tsp ground cumin
- 6 cups cooked red kidney beans
- 4 tbsps olive oil
- 2 yellow onions, chopped
- 4 carrots, sliced
- 3 cups vegetable broth
- 2 tsps ras el hanout
- 4 russet potatoes, chopped
- 2 (29-oz) can crushed tomatoes
- 2 (8-oz) cans diced green chilies, drained

Procedure:

1. First, heat the oil in a pot over medium heat.
2. Place the onion, garlic, ginger, and carrots and sauté for 5 minutes until tender.
3. Then stir in cumin, ras el hanout, potatoes, beans, tomatoes, chiles, and broth.

4. Now season with salt and pepper.
5. Bring to a boil, then lower the heat and simmer for 20 minutes.
6. Add in eggplants and cook for 10 minutes.
7. Serve garnished with peanuts.

Easy Pearl Barley & Vegetable Stew

Servings: 12

Preparation Time: 30 minutes

Ingredients:

- 6 tbsps olive oil
- 2 cups pearl barley
- 4 turnips, chopped
- 8 potatoes, chopped
- 2 (56-oz) can diced tomatoes
- 6 tsps dried mixed herbs
- Salt and black pepper to taste
- 2 onions, chopped
- 4 garlic cloves, minced

Procedure:

1. First of all, warm oil in a pot over medium heat.
2. Then add onion and garlic and sauté for 3 minutes until fragrant. Stir in the turnips, potatoes, barley, tomatoes, 6 cups water, and herbs.
3. Now cook for 20 minutes. Serve.

Homemade Vegetable Chili

Servings: 8

Preparation Time: 30 minutes

Ingredients:

- 4 garlic cloves, minced
- 2 potatoes, cubed
- 2 tbsps tomato paste
- 2 (28-oz) cans of chickpeas
- 2 onions, chopped
- 2 cups vegetable broth
- 2 tsps chili powder
- 2 carrots, chopped
- 4 tsp olive oil
- 2 (56-oz) cans of tomatoes
- Salt and black pepper to taste
- 1/2 cup parsley leaves, chopped

Procedure:

1. First, heat oil in a pot over medium heat.
2. Place in onion and garlic and sauté for 3 minutes.
3. Then add in potato, carrot, tomatoes, broth, tomato paste, chickpeas, and chili; season. Simmer for 20 minutes.
4. Serve garnished with parsley.

Easy Chili Gazpacho

Servings: 8

Preparation Time: 15 minutes

Ingredients:

- 12 tomatoes, chopped
- 2 red bell peppers, diced
- 4 garlic cloves, minced
- 4 tbsps olive oil
- 4 cups water
- 1 tsp chili pepper
- 2 red onions, chopped
- Juice of e lemons
- 4 tbsps chopped fresh basil

Procedure:

1. Take a food processor, place the olive oil, half of the onion, half of the tomato, half of the bell pepper, garlic, lemon juice, basil, and chili pepper.
2. Season with salt and pepper.
3. Blitz until smooth.
4. Transfer to a bowl and add in the reserved onion, tomatoes, and bell pepper.
5. Let chill in the fridge before serving.

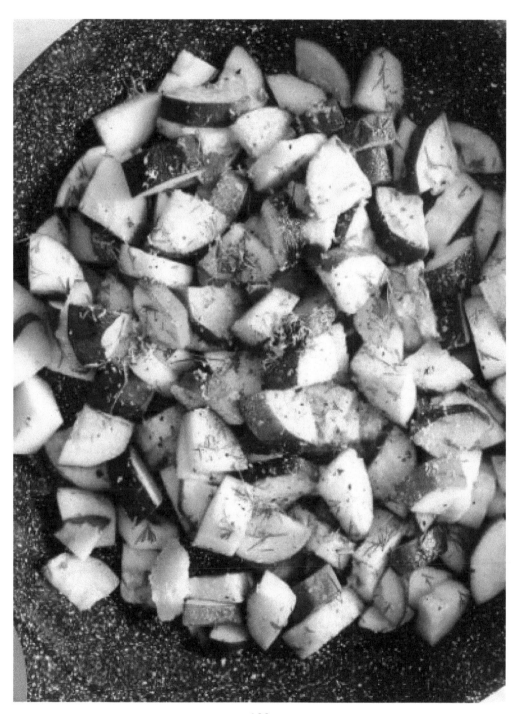

Zucchini Skillet

Servings: 8

Preparation Time: 10 minutes

Per Serving: Calories: 137; Fat: 6.7g; Carbs: 13.2g; Protein: 7.7g

Ingredients:

- 1 teaspoon dried thyme
- 1 teaspoon celery seeds
- 2 teaspoons garlic, minced
- 3 pounds zucchini, sliced
- Flaky sea salt and ground black pepper, to taste
- 2 teaspoons paprika
- 4 tablespoons vegan butter
- 2 shallots, thinly sliced
- 1 teaspoon cayenne pepper
- 1 teaspoon coriander pepper
- 4 tablespoons nutritional yeast

Procedure:

1. Take a saucepan, melt the vegan butter over medium-high heat.
2. Once hot, sauté the shallot for about 3 minutes or until tender. Then, sauté the garlic for about 1 minute until aromatic.
3. Then add in the zucchini, along with the spices, and continue to sauté for 6 minutes more until tender.
4. Finally, taste and adjust the seasonings. Top with nutritional yeast and serve.

Sherry Roasted King Trumpet

Servings: 8

Preparation Time: 20 minutes

Per Serving: Calories: 138; Fat: 7.8g; Carbs: 11.8g; Protein: 5.7g

Ingredients:

- 3 pounds king trumpet mushrooms, cleaned and sliced in half lengthwise.
- 1 teaspoon dried thyme
- 1 teaspoon dried parsley flakes
- 2 teaspoons Dijon mustard
- 4 tablespoons olive oil
- 8 cloves of garlic, minced or chopped
- 1 teaspoon dried rosemary
- 1/2 cup dry sherry
- Sea salt and freshly ground black pepper, to taste

Procedure:

1. First, start by preheating your oven to 390 degrees F. Line a large baking pan with parchment paper.
2. Take a mixing bowl, toss the mushrooms with the remaining ingredients until well coated on all sides.

3. Then place the mushrooms in a single layer on the prepared baking pan.
4. Roast the mushrooms for approximately 20 minutes, tossing them halfway through the cooking.

Healthy Beetroot & Potato Puree

Servings: 10

Preparation Time: 35 minutes

Per Serving: Calories: 177; Fat: 5.6g; Carbs: 28.2g; Protein: 4g

Ingredients:

- 4 tablespoons vegan butter
- 1 teaspoon deli mustard
- 1 cup soy milk
- 3 pounds potatoes, peeled and diced
- 2 pounds beetroot, peeled and diced
- 1 teaspoon ground cumin
- 2 teaspoons paprika
- Sea salt and ground black pepper, to taste

Procedure:

1. First, cook the potatoes and beetroot in boiling salted water until they've softened, about 30 minutes; drain.
2. Then puree the vegetables with vegan butter, mustard, milk, cumin, paprika, salt, and black pepper to your desired consistency.

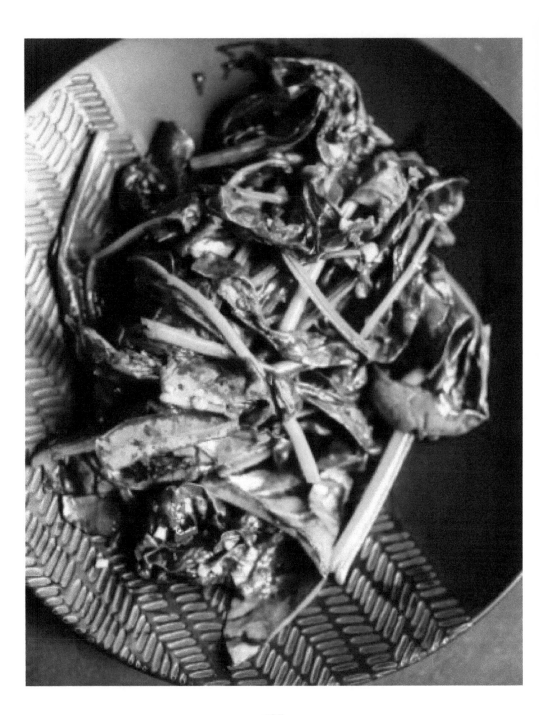

Stir-Fried Thai Spinach

Servings: 8

Preparation Time: 15 minutes

Per Serving: Calories: 147; Fat: 8.9g; Carbs: 12.7g; Protein: 7.1g

Ingredients:

- 2 Bird's eye chili peppers, minced
- 4 cloves of garlic, minced
- 3 pounds spinach leaves, torn into pieces
- 1/2 cup vegetable broth
- 4 tablespoons sesame oil
- 2 onions, chopped
- 2 carrots, trimmed and chopped
- 1/4 cup coconut milk, unsweetened

Procedure:

1. Take a saucepan, heat the sesame oil over medium-high heat.
2. Then, sauté the onion and carrot for about 3 minutes or until tender.
3. Then, sauté the garlic and Bird's eye chili for about 1 minute until aromatic.
4. Now add in the broth and spinach and bring to a boil.

5. Turn the heat to a simmer and continue to cook for 5 minutes longer.
6. Add in the coconut milk and simmer for a further 5 minutes or until everything is cooked

Roasted Squash Mash

Servings: 10

Preparation Time: 35 minutes

Per Serving: Calories: 157; Fat: 5.7g; Carbs: 27g; Protein: 1.7g

Ingredients:

- 4 tablespoons olive oil
- 1 teaspoon garlic powder
- Sea salt and ground black pepper, to taste
- A pinch of grated nutmeg
- A pinch of kosher salt
- 4 tablespoons agave nectar
- 1 teaspoon mustard seeds
- 1 teaspoon celery seeds
- 4 pounds butternut squash

Procedure:

1. First, start by preheating your oven to 420 degrees F.
2. Toss the squash with the remaining ingredients.
3. Then roast the butternut squash for about 30 minutes or until tender and caramelized.
4. Then, in your food processor or blender, puree the roasted squash along with the remaining ingredients until uniform and smooth.

Lightning Source UK Ltd.
Milton Keynes UK
UKHW021816160421
382089UK00001B/59